BRAIN LANGUAGE DICTIONARY

Decoding The Brain Made Easy.

DAVID GOMADZA

FIRST PRESIDENT OF THE WORLD

ISBN: 978-1-4477-5106-9

Brain Language Dictionary

DEDICATION

To the most technologically advanced stage in human development.

This book is part of the Thoughts to Word or Audio series.

This is Volume VII
This book must be used with all the books and is part of the books
and the patents.

ISBN-13: 979-8703923498

https://play.google.com/store/books/details/David_Gomadza_Tho
ughts_To_Word_Or_Audio?id=q2xmEAAAQBAJ&gl=GB

Use The Brain language Construction Rules in All the Books in The Series.

The Golden Rule: The 7 Expressions of Every Word on Earth.

Every word on earth must have a minimum of seven expressions, forms, and definitions. The brain stores words in four sections of the brain. The front right side, the front left side, the right back side, and the left back side. Words used every day are stored in the right back side of the brain. But this depends on the people and geographical regions among other things. For this book and the Thoughts to Word or audio, we will use the right back side as the main region for everyday speech.

But there are other words like those to do with women; she, her, wife, mother, herself, knickers, dress, etc and everything divine; God, Jesus, angels, evil, demons, etc these words are stored in the left back side of the brain or LBS. But words like President [myself] and government are stored on top middle part of the brain. This might be due to evolution.

One must also know that the brain stores other words not in the brain but in the organs or parts defining these words. Legs, hands, etc are stored in specific parts of the body. Again, this just depends on the person concerned.

The body stores the alphabetical order on the body from the collarbone going down to the feet.

So, the brain language as the beginning of a sequence, points to the place in which the brain stores the word. So, if it is in the right back side then we can construct the language as below.

Let us take the word; brain for example.

Right Back Side [RBS] + B+R+A+I+N

So, in the brain language construction sequence the brain points to the place the word brain is stored, RBS. Plus, the place in the body where all the letters are stored that make up that word. Check the alphabetical order of the brain in Brain Code.

https://play.google.com/store/books/details/David_Gomadza_Brain_Code_The_Benchmark_of_Decoding?id=50a3EAAAQBAJ&gl=GB

So, every brain language sequence or sentence starts with a Start.

A position on the brain where the word is stored which acts as a reference point.

But just like in the English language, the sentence must end with a full stop.

To the brain, it must also end all sentences and actions. So, it does this with a deflation state. A return to the initial position. A calm state. This is because the language of the brain is composed of vibrations and movements. So, after all the vibrations and movements, the Deflate position acts as an end to all these vibrations and movements. This is the 'full stop' of every sentence. Now let us see our example above.

Brain.

RBS+B+R+A+I+N+D where D is the Deflate state.

This is the brain language sequence.

So, if a person thinks about the word brain as part of the 7-expression golden rule. The programming language or algorithm or Deep learning AI must create the sequence by pointing at the places on the body where all the sequence letters are. On a robot [Ones I am going to make] the AI software must point to the Right Back Side of the brain. The place on the body where B, R, A, I, and N are stored. To finish the sequence must include a Deflate reference. Once the sequence is completed this trigger all the seven other forms to spell that sequencing in their own expression language; that is either EEG, fMRI, MEG scans or spectrograms, sound waves, acoustic waves etc. So, in the English language the word brain, might pop up on the screen of a translator that is synchronised to this robot or person.

The acoustic machine will produce the acoustic version of the word Brain. The EEG, MEG, PET, and fMRI encoders must receive the sequence as well and produce the spectrogram, scans, etc.

A computer synchronized to this robot must produce the binary value of the word brain at the same time.

In the end, as everything must be synchronized, you will end up with seven different meanings of the word brain at the same time.

A neural network with seven terminals as input is to be used. The seven terminals are used to collect different expressions of the word brain. Then all the information is sent to three decoding points. Where all are analysed and compared. Once the meaning is clear that it is that of the word brain. Then the information is sent to a point where the user knows that the person was thinking about the word brain.

The GREATEST breakthrough of the century.

Visit www.twofuture.world

Signed David Gomadza

First Global President of the World

Brain Language Dictionary

ACKNOWLEDGMENTS

We must all work smarter and harder to better humanity.

Flowers	Right Back Side	Back right head. Dimples. Smile.
Book	Right Back Side	Both arms open outward. Both arms open outward. Left eye. Right eye. Nose bridge downward.
Shadow	Right Back Side	Lean back and back to centre. Deflates.
Shake	Right Back Side	Right ear vibrations. Move waistline to right. Move waistline to left. Slide hand at waistline to right.
Was	Right Back Side	Turn head left from centre. Turn head right. Centre. Throat and downward motion. Shoulders down.
Smiles	Right Back Side	Actual mouth and facial movements.
Hair	Right Back Side	All area covered by hair.
Hot	Right Back Side	Back left shoulder drops.

It	Right Back Side	Back right hand. Downward motion.
Cold	Right Back Side	Back right shoulder drops.
Eagle	Left Back Side	Back right wing. Left back wing. Centre and downward motion. Bend down. Right leg. Left leg. Centre.
Of	Left Back Side	Back top left shoulder click. Deflates.
To	Right Back Side	Back top right shoulder click. Deflates.
Divide	Right Back Side	Backward slanting backward. Deflates.
Tree	Right Back Side	Backward slanting. Forward slanting. Deflates.
Within	Right Back Side	Below chest nudge. Click.
Eight	Right Front	Below left chest. Downward motion.
Seven	Left Front	Below right chest. Downward motion.

Abacus	Right Back Side	Bend at waist front
About	Right Back Side	Bend at waist tilted to left side of body. looking left
Abash	Right Back Side	Bend down between chest and stomach. Straight again.
Squat	Right Back Side	Bend knees. Back to position. Drop shoulders.
Abandonment	Right Back Side	Body drifting sideways left to right like e tree in wind.
Bird	Right Back Side	Both arms open outwards. Downward motion. Drop shoulder.
Amplify	Right Back Side	Both hands open in an outward motion. Top left shoulder click. Right top shoulder. Deflates down.
Down	Right Back Side	Both shoulders down. Both up slightly. Both down to bottom.
Up	Left Back Side	Both shoulders up. Both shoulders down.
Abbreviate	Right Back Side	Bottom Lip. Top lip. Bottom lip. Top lip.

Account	Left Back Side	Left side 45 degrees head turn. [Same to right side] Twice turn head to left. Once to right. Turn head left 45 degrees twice.
Victory	Right Back Side	Chest circular motion. Downward motion. Deflates.
absolute	Right Back Side	Chest out. Chest back. All three times
Big	Right Back Side	Circle face. Outward spiral.
bottom	Right Back Side	Circle motion at foot level right to left.
Like	Right Back Side	Circle mouth. Deflates.
middle	Right Back Side	Circle waist area right to left. Centre front. Downward motion to ground.
Amen	Left Back Side	Circular motion above eyes. Centre neck and downward.
Morning	Right Back Side	Circular motion around chest.
Daughter	Left Back Side	Circular motion around chest. Downward motion.

After	Right Back Side	Circular motion around the waist. Deflates.
Evening	Left Back Side	Circular motion in middle of stomach. Centre stomach. Deflates.
God	Left Back Side	Circular motion round a crown. Centre of face downward. Right chest. Left chest. Bend down seven times. Right chest. Deflate.
Stomach	Right Back Side	Circular pointing to stomach. Deflates.
Close door	Right Back Side	Close mouth. Left chest deflates.
A	Right Back Side	Collar bone
Aback	Right Back Side	Collar bone. Left hip bone
Abort	Right Back Side	Deflate. Turn left. Turn right.
Abandon	Right Back Side	Deflated down
abandoned	Right Back Side	Deflated down

Slow down	Right Back Side	Deflates back heavy then to left.
Demon	Left Back Side	Fast circular motion around eyes.
Between	Right Back Side	Front groin.
Abroad	Right Back Side	Front left shoulder right round to back shoulder and back. Same right shoulder.
Abdicate	Right Back Side	gentle head shake left right left right
Strong	Right Back Side	Hands bulges both sides. Deflates.
Cuddle	Right Back Side	Hands hugging body.
abduct	Right Back Side	Head 180 degrees turn to left side.
Abe	Right Back Side	Head tilt to left
Abhor	Right Back Side	Head tilt to left

Abstain	Right Back Side	Head tilts left and back.
Abuse	Right Back Side	Head turn 45 degrees to left six times. Then to centre. Turn 45 degrees to left. Raise body up.
Absurd	Right Back Side	Head turn left twice. Head turn right twice.
Abnormal	Right Back Side	Head turn right. Head turn left. Deflate.
Angels	Left Back Side	Holy crown. Downward motion. Bend down and back.
Question	Right Back Side	Inside left-hand centre. Thumb. Inside right hand. Right thumb. Centre chest and downward motion.
This	Right Back Side	Inside left-hand palm. Shoulder drops.
Accident	Right Back Side	Jerk forward. Look left. Look right. Slump down.
To	Right Back Side	Left back head. Downward motion. Deflates.
Accomplice	Right Back Side	Left back side of the brain. Head turn backwards to left and back.

Good	Right Back Side	Left centre chest. Deflates.
End	Right Back Side	Left centre chest. Middle of body below chest.
Evil	Left Back Side	Left centre chest. Switching off click. Deflates.
Stay	Right Back Side	Left chest. Bend at waist and back straight.
Please	Right Back Side	Left chest. Bend down. Back straight. Shoulders down Bend.
Wife	Left Back Side	Left chest. Centre of chest downward motion. Top left shoulder. Downward motion. Deflates.
Today	Left Back Side	Left chest. Downward motion from this side. Deflates.
Me	Right Back Side	Left chest. Downward motion. Deflates.
Male	Right Back Side	Left chest. Genitals. Deflates.
Four	Left Front	Left chest. Right chest. Left chest. Downward motion.

Brother	Right Back Side	Left chest. Right chest. Middle of the body below chest. Downward motion.
Two	Right Front	Left chest. Right chest. Right chest downward motion.
When	Left Back Side	Left ear vibrations. Bend at waist to left side.
Who	Right Back Side	Left ear vibrations. Bend at waist to left side.
Was	Left Back Side	Left ear vibrations. Bend to left at waist.
test	Right Back Side	Left ear vibrations. Right ear vibrations. Slide to the left side.
Power off	Right Back Side	Left ear. Left chest. Move to right.
Hie	Left Back Side	Left ear. Right ear. Left chest. Chest deflates.
Analyse	Right Back Side	Left ear. Right ear. Nose bridge all way down.
Sleep	Right Back Side	Left eye to right eye. Ove waist out to left. Learn right.

Warning	Right Back Side	Left eye to right eye. Right eye. Centre. Deflates down.
Vision	Left Back Side	Left eye. Right eye. Node bridge down. Centre chest downward. Shoulders deflates.
Sun	Right Back Side	Left eye. Right eye. Right dimple. Left dimple. Right cheek movement. Left cheek movement. Mouth open. Deflates.
Degrees	Right Back Side	Left head side. 360 rotations. Deflates. Middle of body downward motion. Deflates.
Remote	Right Back Side	Left nipple. Fast deflate to left.
Change	Right Back Side	Left nipple. Rotate 45 degrees.
Year	Right Back Side	Left right top shoulder. Right top shoulder. Spiral downward. Bottom left foot. Bottom right leg. Top neck downward movement.
Back	Right Back Side	Left shoulder to right shoulder. Right shoulder to left shoulder. Middle of chest and move down.
Yes	Right Back Side	Left shoulder. Right shoulder. Right waist. Left waist. Deflates.
Ok	Right Back Side	Left shoulder. Right waist. Left waist.

Repeat	Right Back Side	Left shoulder. Right waist. Left waist. Deflate.
Stop	Right Back Side	Left shoulder. Turn left 90 degrees. Look front. Slide to left and back. Stop. Deflate.
Cherubim	Left Back Side	Left side brain. Right top back shoulder. Left top shoulder. Neck downward motion. Imitate flying. Open wings twice. Deflates.
Woman	Left Back Side	Left side just below left chest. [Top rib]
Accommodate	Right Back Side	Left side of the brain.
Look left	Right Back Side	Left side of the brain. Left eye. Turn left at waist.
Weak	Right Back Side	Left side on brain. Bend down.
Add	Right Back Side	Left side top front shoulder. Right side top shoulder. Left side waist. Right side waist. Left side knee. Right side knee. Left side ankle. Right side ankle. Neck going down.
Choose	Right Back Side	Left side top hand. Circular motion at waist. Downward motion. Deflates.

Abortion	Right Back Side	Left stomach. Head turn left side.
Plastic	Right Back Side	Left top brain side. Turn to right. Turn to left. Back centre.
One	Right Back Side	Left top collarbone. Downward motion. Deflates.
There	Right Back Side	Left top collarbone. Downward motion. Deflates.
abaft	Right Back Side	left top shoulder. Bend at waist to right side.
Abridge	Right Back Side	Left top shoulder. Right top shoulder. Shoulders down.
Beside	Right Back Side	Left top shoulder. Rotate right to left 45 degrees. Deflate.
Month	Left Back Side	Left top shoulder. Right top shoulder. Spiral movement down centre body. Cortex. Below left foot. Below right foot. Deflates.
Give	Right Back Side	Lift left hand outward.
From	Right Back Side	Lift right hand outward. Lift left hand outward.

That	Right Back Side	Lift right hand outward. Lift left hand outward.
aboard	Right Back Side	Lift right hand. Lift left hand.
Lion	Right Back Side	Long right jaw. Long left jaw. Mouth wide open. Bend to a four-legged animal. Right front paw. Left front paw. Right back leg. Left back leg. Tail. Deflates.
Access	Right Back Side	Look left twice. Lift body up. Look left twice.
Accelerate	Right Back Side	Look over to left. Look over to right. Twice. Look forward. Lift chest up.
Fast	Right Back Side	Lower back neck vibrations. Drop down shoulders fast.
I kiss you	Right Back Side	Lower lip. Upper lip [mouth]. Left chest. Right chest. Deflates.
Accent	Right Back Side	Lower lip. Upper lip. Lower lip. Upper lip. Drop right shoulder.
Day	Left Back Side	Middle of neck. Turn 45 degrees left to right. Then right to left. Downward motion.
Break	Right Back Side	Middle of the body below chest. Breaks

Pause	Right Back Side	Middle of the body below chest. Vibrates.
Nine	Right Front	Middle of the chest. Left hand side of body below left chest. Downward motion.
Milk	Right Back Side	Mouth drinking motion. Stomach. Right breast. Left breast. Centre of body downward. Deflates.
Eat	Right Back Side	Mouth open. Food down. To stomach. Out. Deflates.
Ask	Right Back Side	Mouth opens wide. Both cheeks closes.
Channel	Left Back Side	Mouth vibrations.
Keep	Right Back Side	Move right to left. Centre again. Shoulders down.
Air	Right Back Side	Movement in nostrils. Throat. Lungs. Circulate body and out.
Spine	Right Back Side	Neck down.
Computer	Right Back Side	Neck tightening. Back shoulder deflates. Bending down.

Shirt	Right Back Side	Neck. Spiral down to waist. Downward motion.
Inflate	Right Back Side	Nostril. Waist move left side lean right.
Powerful	Right Back Side	Open arms fast wide.
Sight	Right Back Side	Open mouth. Deflates.
Open door	Right Back Side	Open mouth. Left chest deflates.
Loose	Right Back Side	Orifice. Deflates.
Lick	Right Back Side	Point of lick. Deflate waistline.
Hair	Right Back Side	Point to actual parts of the body.
News	Right Back Side	Point to right ear. Point to left ear. Right top shoulder. Left top shoulder. Centre chest. All way down. Drop shoulders.
Ribs	Right Back Side	Pointing to three parts of ribs

Blood	Right Back Side	Pointing to all parts with blood.
Clothes	Right Back Side	Points to all places covered by cloths.
Overtake	Right Back Side	Push right chest forward.
Gun	Right Back Side	Right hand. Inside hand. Backward motion. Forward motion.
Breath in	Right Back Side	Right ear vibrations. Inflate. Stomach in.
Next	Right Back Side	Right back elbow. Bend forward.
Click	Right Back Side	Right back head side. Soft deflates.
Label	Right Back Side	Right back head. Downward motion. Deflates.
From	Right Back Side	Right back shoulder. Left back shoulder. Downward motion. Deflates.
Jacket	Right Back Side	Right back shoulder. Left back shoulder. Front neck. Downward motion.

Code	Right Back Side	Right back top shoulder. Right side deflates.
Ox	Right Back Side	Right back. Left back. Right back near tail. Left back near tail. Bend down. Front right leg. Front left leg. Back right leg. Back left leg. Tail. Back to centre position. Bellows.
Shut down	Right Back Side	Right bottom neck soft bending. Left stomach deflate.
Female	Left Back Side	Right breast. Left breast. Front genital. Deflates.
Time	Right Back Side	Right centre chest. Right hand wrist. Left hand wrist. Downward motion.
Together	Right Back Side	Right check. Left check. Right chest. Deflates.
Accelerate	Right Back Side	Right chest fast.
Tomorrow	Right Back Side	Right chest side. Downward motion on this side. Deflates.
For	Right Back Side	Right chest. Downward motion.

Add	Right Back Side	Right chest. Horizontal motion. Left chest. Reverse horizontal motion. Right chest. Top chest to downward motion. Deflates.
Five	Right Back Side	Right chest. Below right chest. Downward motion.
Abase	Right Back Side	Right Chest. Bends at waist.
Yesterday	Right Back Side	Right chest. Breaks
Abreast	Right Back Side	Right chest. Chest out. Chest back.
End	Right Back Side	Right chest. Click. Deflates.
Abide	Right Back Side	Right Chest. Deflate. Lift right hand.
Husband	Right Back Side	Right chest. Downward motion.
Want	Right Back Side	Right chest. Downward motion.
Genesis	Right Back Side	Right chest. Downward motion. Deflates.

Win	Right Back Side	Right chest. Downward motion. Deflates.
Jesus	Left Back Side	Right chest. Left chest. Bend down. Right chest downward motion. Deflates.
Chest	Right Back Side	Right chest. Left chest. Deflates.
Internet	Right Back Side	Right chest. Left chest. Deflates.
Begin	Right Back Side	Right chest. Left chest. Left chest downward motion. Deflates.
Count	Right Back Side	Right chest. Left chest. Middle of body and downward.
Calculate	Right Back Side	Right chest. Left chest. Middle of body just below chest.
Sister	Left Back Side	Right chest. Left chest. Middle of the body below chest. Downward motion.
Three	Right Back Side	Right chest. Left chest. Below right chest. Downward motion. Deflates.
Six	Right Back Side	Right chest. Middle of body below chest. Downward motion.

Reduce speed	Right Back Side	Right chest. Slow downward motion.
Fight	Right Back Side	Right chest. Turn to right. Turn left.
End	Right Back Side	Right ear vibrations. Gentle turn left.
Breath out	Right Back Side	Right ear vibrations. Deflate. Stomach out.
Believe	Right Back Side	Right ear vibrations. Left chest deflates. Slide waist to right. Slide to left. Centre.
I	Right Back Side	Right ear vibrations. Bend back outwards waist level.
Park	Right Back Side	Right ear Vibrate. Deflect bending down outward.
Or	Right Back Side	Right ear vibrations.
Play	Right Back Side	Right ear vibrations. Turn head left. Left nipple. Shoulders slump.
Sit	Right Back Side	Right ear vibrations. Actual sitting. Bending down bending knees.

U-turn	Right Back Side	Right ear vibrations. Anticlockwise turn.
Reverse	Right Back Side	Right ear vibrations. Deflates bending down outward.
Am	Right Back Side	Right ear vibrations. Deflates down fast.
The	Right Back Side	Right ear vibrations. Gently turn right.
Listen	Right Back Side	Right ear vibrations. Left chest deep deflate. Drop shoulders.
Deflate	Right Back Side	Right ear vibrations. Left chest deflates. Move waist level to left. Move waist to right. Right back shoulder. Centre middle shoulder. Downward motion.
President	Centre Top Brain	Right ear vibrations. Left chest deflates. Move waist level to left. Move waist to right. Right back shoulder. Centre middle shoulder. Downward motion.
At	Right Back Side	Right ear vibrations. Left ear vibrations. Lower lip. Upper lip. Drag top lip down.
Tell	Right Back Side	Right ear vibrations. Left ear vibrations. Lower lip. Upper lip. Drag top lip down.

Sing	Right Back Side	Right ear vibrations. Left ear. Outpouring of emotions in left chest.
Run	Right Back Side	Right ear vibrations. Left leg. Right leg. Under foot tapping's.
Do	Right Back Side	Right ear vibrations. Left side rib. Slide to left.
Horn	Right Back Side	Right ear vibrations. Lower left stomach.
Man	Right Back Side	Right ear vibrations. Middle point of body just below the chest.
Dollars	Right Back Side	Right ear vibrations. Right eye. Downward motion. Shoulders down.
Radio	Right Back Side	Right ear vibrations. Right nipple. Deflate fast.
Command	Right Back Side	Right ear vibrations. Slide to left. Slide to right at waist level. Slide to left side.
Go	Right Back Side	Right ear. Bed backward.
You	Right Back Side	Right ear. Deflates.

Yours	Right Back Side	Right ear. Deflates.
Close window	Right Back Side	Right ear. Drop shoulders down.
Drive	Right Back Side	Right ear. Left chest vibrations. Slide hand to right side.
Accept	Right Back Side	Right ear. Left chest. Slide outward to left.
Horn	Right Back Side	Right ear. Left ear vibrations.
Beep	Left Back Side	Right ear. Left ear. Armpit vibrations.
Talk	Right Back Side	Right ear. Left ear. Left chest. Deflates
Power on	Right Back Side	Right ear. Left ear. Right chest., Left chest. Deflates.
Glasses	Right Back Side	Right ear. Left ear. Right eye. Left eye. Nose bridge. Downward
Ask	Right Back Side	Right ear. Left ear. Slide left line to right.

Beg	Right Back Side	Right ear. Left ear. Slide left. Bend backward.
Open	Right Back Side	Right ear. Left ear. Slide to left outside.
Touch	Right Back Side	Right ear. Right hand. Handle.
Donate	Right Back Side	Right ear. Slide to left at waistline.
Follow	Right Back Side	Right ear. Slide to left at waistline. Slide backwards. Lean forward.
Close	Right Back Side	Right ear. Slide to right at waistline.
Moon	Right Back Side	Right ear. Deflates.
Come	Right Back Side	Right ear. Left ear. Bend backward.
Join hands	Right Back Side	Right elbow. Left elbow.
Clap	Right Back Side	Right elbow. Left elbow. Centre hands. Sound and downward motion of sound to ground. Drop shoulder.

Sex	Right Back Side	Right elbow. Left elbow. Front genital. Back orifice. Mouth. Deflates.
Awake	Right Back Side	Right eye to left eye. Move waist to right.
Fish	Right Back Side	Right eye. Bend down. Move lateral. Left. Right. Centre. Tail.
Avoid	Right Back Side	Right eye. Head move left and right. Centre chest downward motion.
Animal	Right Back Side	Right eye. Left eye. Bend Down to a four legged. Right front leg. Left from leg. Right back leg. Left back leg. Tail Straight.
Write	Right Back Side	Right eye. Left eye. Index finger. Left chest. Deflates.
Real	Right Back Side	Right eye. Left eye. Left chest. Deflates.
Beauty	Right Back Side	Right eye. Left eye. Left side cheek smile movement. Left eye soft wink. Deflates.
Trance	Right Back Side	Right eye. Left eye. Pull down face fast. Slump.
Left	Right Back Side	Right eye. Left eye. Right chest. Slide waist to right. Then left.

Mirror	Right Back Side	Right eye. Left eye. Rotate right to left. Left eye. Right eye. Deflate. Drop shoulders.
Left eye	Right Back Side	Right eye. Left eye. Slide right at waist. Slide to left at waist.
Foot	Right Back Side	Right feet. Left feet Centre body. D deflates down
Enter	Right Back Side	Right hand muscle click.
Command	Right Back Side	Right hand shoulder down.
Choice	Right Back Side	Right hand top hand. Left hand top hand. Circular motion at waist. Downward motion. Deflate.
Abattoir	Right Back Side	Right hand top shoulder.
Watch	Right Back Side	Right hand wrist position. Deflates
Which	Right Back Side	Right head side. Bend backward. Centre.
Forward	Right Back Side	Right hand elbow. Vibrations. Bend down backward. Lean forward.

Knee	Right Back Side	Right knee. Left knee. Centre body deflates.
Standing	Right Back Side	Right leg below foot. Left leg below foot. Shoulders drops.
Legs	Right Back Side	Right leg. Left leg.
Walk	Right Back Side	Right leg. Left leg. Drop shoulders.
Switch	Right Back Side	Right nipple. Downward motion. Deflates.
Dance	Right Back Side	Right shoulder. Left shoulder. Right waist. Left waist. Right foot bottom. Left foot bottom. Circular motion on ground. Deflates.
Low	Right Back Side	Right shoulder down
abalone	Right Back Side	Right shoulder down head tilting right
front	Right Back Side	Right shoulder to left shoulder. Left shoulder to right shoulder. Middle chest and down
High	Right Back Side	Right shoulder up. Left shoulder down.

Abrupt	Right Back Side	Right shoulder. Fast right shoulder down.
No	Right Back Side	Right shoulder. Left shoulder. Right waist. Left waist. Deflates.
Start	Right Back Side	Right shoulder. Deflate down.
Father	Right Back Side	Right side of body below right chest. Left chest. Deep deflates.
Lose	Right Back Side	Right side of brain. Downward motion. Deflates.
Absorb	Right Back Side	Right side of the brain.
Danger	Right Back Side	Right side of the brain. Imitate neck break. Centre chest downward motion. Deflates.
abate	Right Back Side	Right side top back shoulder
Metre	Right Back Side	Right to left measurement of a mitre.
achieve	Right Back Side	Right top back shoulder. Left top back shoulder. Centre spine back and all way down.

Paper	Right Back Side	Right top brain side. Turn to left. Turn to right. Back at centre.
The	Right Back Side	Right top collarbone. Downward motion. Deflates.
As	Right Back Side	Right top front forehead. Centre of head and downward.
Tree of life	Left Back Side	Right top shoulder. Left top shoulder Deflates.
Month	Right Back Side	Right top shoulder. Left top shoulder. Left wristwatch-area. Right wristwatch-area. Downward motion.
Is	Right Back Side	Right upper hand near shoulder. Open right hand outward. Deflates.
Turn right	Right Back Side	Rotate left to right 45 degrees.
Rotate	Right Back Side	Rotate right to left 360 degrees.
Turn left	Right Back Side	Rotate right to left 45 degrees.
To	Right Back Side	Rotate round left to right. Drop shoulders.

Heaven	Left Back Side	Rotational motion on top of head right to left right round. Right top shoulder. Left top shoulder. Nose bridge all downward. Bend down backward. Centre. Drop shoulders.
Observe	Right Back Side	See with left eye. See with right eye. Downward movement middle of eye and nose bridge. Right cheek poke. Bend down backward. Straight back.
How	Right Back Side	Shoulders move inwards.
accountable	Right Back Side	Slowly in circular form turn head to left. 90 degrees. Back at centre. From centre turn head right 90 degrees. To centre. Repeat two more times.
Why	Right Back Side	Slowly shake head sideways. Bend forward at waist.
absence	Right Back Side	Slowly turn head left three times.
accrue	Right Back Side	Slowly turn to move head from centre to 45 degrees to left. Then look all the way down. Reverse to centre. Same to right side. Twice.
abundance	Right Back Side	smoothly body turns left then right drifting down

able	Right Back Side	Soft head node.
Fingers	Right Back Side	Start counting from left hand thumb all ten.
abdomen	Right Back Side	Stomach in showing in circular motion
abolish	Right Back Side	Tilt body to left. Tilt body to right. Tilt body to left.
acclaim	Right Back Side	Tilt head 45 degrees to the left. Look right in front. Look 45 degrees down.
Ten	Right Front	Top centre of chest. Down middle of body below chest. Downward motion.
Trinity	Left Back Side	Top forehead. Groin region. Centre chest. Right hand. Left hand. Deflates. Bend down. Centre. Deflates.
Safe	Right Back Side	Top head circular motion. Downward motion. Relax. Shoulders down.
God	Left Back Side	Top head rotation. Top head downward movement. Both shoulders down. Bend down. Right chest. Bend down. Deflates.
Bicycle	Right Back Side	Top head. Turn left and back eight times. One complete revolution. Deflates at centre.

Life	Left Back Side	Top left chest. Centre left chest. Middle of chest downward movement. Deflates.
Second	Right Back Side	Top left shoulder. Bend backward. Back at centre. Drop shoulders.
whistle	Right Back Side	Top lip. Bottom lip. Twist lips and tongue.
Government	Centre top head	Top neck circular motion. Top shoulder circular motion. Middle body circular motion. Knee level circular motion.
Death	Left Back Side	Top neck slight click bend. Head move to left. Middle chest downward motion. Deflates.
First	Right Back Side	Top of head circular motion. Index finger up. Deflates down.
above	Right Back Side	Top of head.
accordance	Right Back Side	Top of head. Bend forward to check. Lift head up. Turn head 45 degrees right. Look straight forward. Turn head 45 degrees left. Look straight ahead. Bend head forward. Back straight.
top	Right Back Side	Top of head. Centre head and downward motion.

Two hundred	Right Front	Top of thumb. First joint of thumb. Deflates.
Three thousand	Left Front	Top of thumb. First joint of thumb. Second joint of thumb.
They	Right Back Side	Top right-hand shoulder. Along arm downward motion. Deflates.
Tonight	Right Back Side	Top right-hand shoulder. Deflates.
Calendar.	Left Back Side	Top right shoulder. Top left shoulder Right lower rib. Left lower rib. Right foot. Left foot. Top of head downward motion to ground.
Holy spirit	Left Back Side	Top shoulder circular motion. Centre. Downward motion. Bend down. Centre.
Year	Right Back Side	Top shoulder circular motion. Centre chest. Downward motion to ground.
Spirit	Left Back Side	Top shoulder circular motion right to left. Centre body downward. Deflates.
One hundred	Right Front	Top thumb. Deflates down.
Always	Right Back Side	Turn 180 degrees from right to left. One complete revolution. Deflates.

Strict	Right Back Side	Turn head 30 degrees from right to left. Back at centre. Deflates
acquire	Right Back Side	Turn head 30 degrees left. Look down in front. Stretch hands to pick up. Lift. Then put down hands.
acid	Right Back Side	Turn head 30 degrees to left. Throw eyes fast. Centre head and repeat five times. Shocked and scared.
accuracy	Right Back Side	Turn head 45 degrees to left. Eyes full beam check everything. Look centre. Do same right side. Look centre. Repeat. Same eyes full beam both sides. Learn forward squint eyes to check. Node head slightly. Repeats everything.
accept	Right Back Side	Turn head 45 degrees.
Subtract	Right Back Side	Turn head from left to right. Right deflates down
Many	Right Back Side	Turn head left to right. Bend down. Shoulder deflates.
where	Right Back Side	Turn head left. Turn head right. Drop shoulders.
Multiply	Right Back Side	Turn head right to left. Left deflates.

who	Right Back Side	Turn head right. Then left. Drop shoulders.
How	Right Back Side	Turn head to left 90 degrees. Centre chest down.
Judgement	Left Back Side	Turn head to left and back. Slowly deflate.
Was	Right Back Side	Turn left from right at waist. Back at centre. Deflates.
Box	Right Back Side	Turn left. Turn right. Centre chest downward.
apologise	Right Back Side	Turn to side. Right chest. Left chest. Deflates
centre	Right Back Side	up and down around genital area.
cry	Right Back Side	Upper face. Bottom face. Downward motion from upper face down.
voice	Right Back Side	Voice box on neck. Right chest. Left chest. Shoulders drops.
Knickers	Left Back Side	Waist circular motion right to left. Groin region. Deflates.

Trousers	Right Back Side	Waist circular motion. Downward.
a	Right Back Side	
able	Right Back Side	
about	Right Back Side	
above	Right Back Side	
act	Right Back Side	

THE BRAIN LANGUAGE DICTIONARY.
SEQUENCE CONSTRUCTION

Flowers	=	Right Back Side	+	Flowers	+ D
Book	=	Right Back Side	+	Book	+ D
Shadow	=	Right Back Side	+	Shadow	+ D
Shake	=	Right Back Side	+	Shake	+ D
Was	=	Right Back Side	+	Was	+ D
Smiles	=	Right Back Side	+	Smiles	+ D
Hair	=	Right Back Side	+	Hair	+ D
Hot	=	Right Back Side	+	Hot	+ D
It	=	Right Back Side	+	It	+ D
Cold	=	Right Back Side	+	Cold	+ D
Eagle	=	Left Back Side	+	Eagle	+ D
Of	=	Left Back Side	+	Of	+ D
To	=	Right Back Side	+	To	+ D
Divide	=	Right Back Side	+	Divide	+ D
Tree	=	Right Back Side	+	Tree	+ D
Within	=	Right Back Side	+	Within	+ D
Eight	=	Right Front	+	Eight	+ D
Seven	=	Left Front	+	Seven	+ D

Abacus	=	Right Back Side	+	Abacus	+	D
About	=	Right Back Side	+	About	+	D
Abash	=	Right Back Side	+	Abash	+	D
Squat	=	Right Back Side	+	Squat	+	D
Abandonment	=	Right Back Side	+	Abandonment	+	D
Bird	=	Right Back Side	+	Bird	+	D
Amplify	=	Right Back Side	+	Amplify	+	D
Down	=	Right Back Side	+	Down	+	D
Up	=	Left Back Side	+	Up	+	D
Abbreviate	=	Right Back Side	+	Abbreviate	+	D
Account	=	Left Back Side	+	Account	+	D
Victory	=	Right Back Side	+	Victory	+	D
absolute	=	Right Back Side	+	absolute	+	D
Big	=	Right Back Side	+	Big	+	D
bottom	=	Right Back Side	+	bottom	+	D
Like	=	Right Back Side	+	Like	+	D
middle	=	Right Back Side	+	middle	+	D
Amen	=	Left Back Side	+	Amen	+	D
Morning	=	Right Back Side	+	Morning	+	D
Daughter	=	Left Back Side	+	Daughter	+	D

After	=	Right Back Side	+	After	+	D
Evening	=	Left Back Side	+	Evening	+	D
God	=	Left Back Side	+	God	+	D
Stomach	=	Right Back Side	+	Stomach	+	D
Close door	=	Right Back Side	+	Close door	+	D
A	=	Right Back Side	+	A	+	D
Aback	=	Right Back Side	+	Aback	+	D
Abort	=	Right Back Side	+	Abort	+	D
Abandon	=	Right Back Side	+	Abandon	+	D
abandoned	=	Right Back Side	+	abandoned	+	D
Slow down	=	Right Back Side	+	Slow down	+	D
Demon	=	Left Back Side	+	Demon	+	D
Between	=	Right Back Side	+	Between	+	D
Abroad	=	Right Back Side	+	Abroad	+	D
Abdicate	=	Right Back Side	+	Abdicate	+	D
Strong	=	Right Back Side	+	Strong	+	D
Cuddle	=	Right Back Side	+	Cuddle	+	D
abduct	=	Right Back Side	+	abduct	+	D
Abe	=	Right Back Side	+	Abe	+	D

Abhor	=	Right Back Side	+	Abhor	+	D
Abstain	=	Right Back Side	+	Abstain	+	D
Abuse	=	Right Back Side	+	Abuse	+	D
Absurd	=	Right Back Side	+	Absurd	+	D
Abnormal	=	Right Back Side	+	Abnormal	+	D
Angels	=	Left Back Side	+	Angels	+	D
Question	=	Right Back Side	+	Question	+	D
This	=	Right Back Side	+	This	+	D
Accident	=	Right Back Side	+	Accident	+	D
To	=	Right Back Side	+	To	+	D
Accomplice	=	Right Back Side	+	Accomplice	+	D
Good	=	Right Back Side	+	Good	+	D
End	=	Right Back Side	+	End	+	D
Evil	=	Left Back Side	+	Evil	+	D
Stay	=	Right Back Side	+	Stay	+	D
Please	=	Right Back Side	+	Please	+	D
Wife	=	Left Back Side	+	Wife	+	D
Today	=	Left Back Side	+	Today	+	D
Me	=	Right Back Side	+	Me	+	D
Male	=	Right Back Side	+	Male	+	D

Four	=	Left Front	+	Four	+ D
Brother	=	Right Back Side	+	Brother	+ D
Two	=	Right Front	+	Two	+ D
When	=	Left Back Side	+	When	+ D
Who	=	Right Back Side	+	Who	+ D
Was	=	Left Back Side	+	Was	+ D
test	=	Right Back Side	+	test	+ D
Power off	=	Right Back Side	+	Power off	+ D
Hie	=	Left Back Side	+	Hie	+ D
Analyse	=	Right Back Side	+	Analyse	+ D
Sleep	=	Right Back Side	+	Sleep	+ D
Warning	=	Right Back Side	+	Warning	+ D
Vision	=	Left Back Side	+	Vision	+ D
Sun	=	Right Back Side	+	Sun	+ D
Degrees	=	Right Back Side	+	Degrees	+ D
Remote	=	Right Back Side	+	Remote	+ D
Change	=	Right Back Side	+	Change	+ D
Year	=	Right Back Side	+	Year	+ D
Back	=	Right Back Side	+	Back	+ D
Yes	=	Right Back Side	+	Yes	+ D
Ok	=	Right Back Side	+	Ok	+ D

Repeat	=	Right Back Side	+	Repeat	+	D
Stop	=	Right Back Side	+	Stop	+	D
Cherubim	=	Left Back Side	+	Cherubim	+	D
Woman	=	Left Back Side	+	Woman	+	D
Accommodate	=	Right Back Side	+	Accommodate	+	D
Look left	=	Right Back Side	+	Look left	+	D
Weak	=	Right Back Side	+	Weak	+	D
Add	=	Right Back Side	+	Add	+	D
Choose	=	Right Back Side	+	Choose	+	D
Abortion	=	Right Back Side	+	Abortion	+	D
Plastic	=	Right Back Side	+	Plastic	+	D
One	=	Right Back Side	+	One	+	D
There	=	Right Back Side	+	There	+	D
abaft	=	Right Back Side	+	abaft	+	D
Abridge	=	Right Back Side	+	Abridge	+	D
Beside	=	Right Back Side	+	Beside	+	D
Month	=	Left Back Side	+	Month	+	D
Give	=	Right Back Side	+	Give	+	D
From	=	Right Back Side	+	From	+	D

That	=	Right Back Side	+	That	+	D
aboard	=	Right Back Side	+	aboard	+	D
Lion	=	Right Back Side	+	Lion	+	D
Access	=	Right Back Side	+	Access	+	D
Accelerate	=	Right Back Side	+	Accelerate	+	D
Fast	=	Right Back Side	+	Fast	+	D
I kiss you	=	Right Back Side	+	I kiss you	+	D
Accent	=	Right Back Side	+	Accent	+	D
Day	=	Left Back Side	+	Day	+	D
Break	=	Right Back Side	+	Break	+	D
Pause	=	Right Back Side	+	Pause	+	D
Nine	=	Right Front	+	Nine	+	D
Milk	=	Right Back Side	+	Milk	+	D
Eat	=	Right Back Side	+	Eat	+	D
Ask	=	Right Back Side	+	Ask	+	D
Channel	=	Left Back Side	+	Channel	+	D
Keep	=	Right Back Side	+	Keep	+	D
Air	=	Right Back Side	+	Air	+	D
Spine	=	Right Back Side	+	Spine	+	D

Computer	=	Right Back Side	+	Computer	+ D
Shirt	=	Right Back Side	+	Shirt	+ D
Inflate	=	Right Back Side	+	Inflate	+ D
Powerful	=	Right Back Side	+	Powerful	+ D
Sight	=	Right Back Side	+	Sight	+ D
Open door	=	Right Back Side	+	Open door	+ D
Loose	=	Right Back Side	+	Loose	+ D
Lick	=	Right Back Side	+	Lick	+ D
Hair	=	Right Back Side	+	Hair	+ D
News	=	Right Back Side	+	News	+ D
Ribs	=	Right Back Side	+	Ribs	+ D
Blood	=	Right Back Side	+	Blood	+ D
Clothes	=	Right Back Side	+	Clothes	+ D
Overtake	=	Right Back Side	+	Overtake	+ D
Gun	=	Right Back Side	+	Gun	+ D
Breath in	=	Right Back Side	+	Breath in	+ D
Next	=	Right Back Side	+	Next	+ D
Click	=	Right Back Side	+	Click	+ D

Label	=	Right Back Side	+	Label	+	D
From	=	Right Back Side	+	From	+	D
Jacket	=	Right Back Side	+	Jacket	+	D
Code	=	Right Back Side	+	Code	+	D
Ox	=	Right Back Side	+	Ox	+	D
Shut down	=	Right Back Side	+	Shut down	+	D
Female	=	Left Back Side	+	Female	+	D
Time	=	Right Back Side	+	Time	+	D
Together	=	Right Back Side	+	Together	+	D
Accelerate	=	Right Back Side	+	Accelerate	+	D
Tomorrow	=	Right Back Side	+	Tomorrow	+	D
For	=	Right Back Side	+	For	+	D
Add	=	Right Back Side	+	Add	+	D
Five	=	Right Back Side	+	Five	+	D
Abase	=	Right Back Side	+	Abase	+	D
Yesterday	=	Right Back Side	+	Yesterday	+	D
Abreast	=	Right Back Side	+	Abreast	+	D
End	=	Right Back Side	+	End	+	D

Abide	=	Right Back Side	+	Abide	+	D
Husband	=	Right Back Side	+	Husband	+	D
Want	=	Right Back Side	+	Want	+	D
Genesis	=	Right Back Side	+	Genesis	+	D
Win	=	Right Back Side	+	Win	+	D
Jesus	=	Left Back Side	+	Jesus	+	D
Chest	=	Right Back Side	+	Chest	+	D
Internet	=	Right Back Side	+	Internet	+	D
Begin	=	Right Back Side	+	Begin	+	D
Count	=	Right Back Side	+	Count	+	D
Calculate	=	Right Back Side	+	Calculate	+	D
Sister	=	Left Back Side	+	Sister	+	D
Three	=	Right Back Side	+	Three	+	D
Six	=	Right Back Side	+	Six	+	D
Reduce speed	=	Right Back Side	+	Reduce speed	+	D
Fight	=	Right Back Side	+	Fight	+	D
End	=	Right Back Side	+	End	+	D
Breath out	=	Right Back Side	+	Breath out	+	D
Believe	=	Right Back Side	+	Believe	+	D

I	=	Right Back Side	+	I	+	D
Park	=	Right Back Side	+	Park	+	D
Or	=	Right Back Side	+	Or	+	D
Play	=	Right Back Side	+	Play	+	D
Sit	=	Right Back Side	+	Sit	+	D
U-turn	=	Right Back Side	+	U-turn	+	D
Reverse	=	Right Back Side	+	Reverse	+	D
Am	=	Right Back Side	+	Am	+	D
The	=	Right Back Side	+	The	+	D
Listen	=	Right Back Side	+	Listen	+	D
Deflate	=	Right Back Side	+	Deflate	+	D
President	=	Centre Top Brain	+	President	+	D
At	=	Right Back Side	+	At	+	D
Tell	=	Right Back Side	+	Tell	+	D
Sing	=	Right Back Side	+	Sing	+	D
Run	=	Right Back Side	+	Run	+	D
Do	=	Right Back Side	+	Do	+	D
Horn	=	Right Back Side	+	Horn	+	D

Man	=	Right Back Side	+	Man	+ D
Dollars	=	Right Back Side	+	Dollars	+ D
Radio	=	Right Back Side	+	Radio	+ D
Command	=	Right Back Side	+	Command	+ D
Go	=	Right Back Side	+	Go	+ D
You	=	Right Back Side	+	You	+ D
Yours	=	Right Back Side	+	Yours	+ D
Close window	=	Right Back Side	+	Close window	+ D
Drive	=	Right Back Side	+	Drive	+ D
Accept	=	Right Back Side	+	Accept	+ D
Horn	=	Right Back Side	+	Horn	+ D
Beep	=	Left Back Side	+	Beep	+ D
Talk	=	Right Back Side	+	Talk	+ D
Power on	=	Right Back Side	+	Power on	+ D
Glasses	=	Right Back Side	+	Glasses	+ D
Ask	=	Right Back Side	+	Ask	+ D
Beg	=	Right Back Side	+	Beg	+ D
Open	=	Right Back Side	+	Open	+ D

Touch	=	Right Back Side	+	Touch	+	D
Donate	=	Right Back Side	+	Donate	+	D
Follow	=	Right Back Side	+	Follow	+	D
Close	=	Right Back Side	+	Close	+	D
Moon	=	Right Back Side	+	Moon	+	D
Come	=	Right Back Side	+	Come	+	D
Join hands	=	Right Back Side	+	Join hands	+	D
Clap	=	Right Back Side	+	Clap	+	D
Sex	=	Right Back Side	+	Sex	+	D
Awake	=	Right Back Side	+	Awake	+	D
Fish	=	Right Back Side	+	Fish	+	D
Avoid	=	Right Back Side	+	Avoid	+	D
Animal	=	Right Back Side	+	Animal	+	D
Write	=	Right Back Side	+	Write	+	D
Real	=	Right Back Side	+	Real	+	D
Beauty	=	Right Back Side	+	Beauty	+	D
Trance	=	Right Back Side	+	Trance	+	D
Left	=	Right Back Side	+	Left	+	D

Mirror	=	Right Back Side	+	Mirror	+	D
Left eye	=	Right Back Side	+	Left eye	+	D
Foot	=	Right Back Side	+	Foot	+	D
Enter	=	Right Back Side	+	Enter	+	D
Command	=	Right Back Side	+	Command	+	D
Choice	=	Right Back Side	+	Choice	+	D
Abattoir	=	Right Back Side	+	Abattoir	+	D
Watch	=	Right Back Side	+	Watch	+	D
Which	=	Right Back Side	+	Which	+	D
Forward	=	Right Back Side	+	Forward	+	D
Knee	=	Right Back Side	+	Knee	+	D
Standing	=	Right Back Side	+	Standing	+	D
Legs	=	Right Back Side	+	Legs	+	D
Walk	=	Right Back Side	+	Walk	+	D
Switch	=	Right Back Side	+	Switch	+	D
Dance	=	Right Back Side	+	Dance	+	D
Low	=	Right Back Side	+	Low	+	D
abalone	=	Right Back Side	+	abalone	+	D

front	=	Right Back Side	+	front	+	D
High	=	Right Back Side	+	High	+	D
Abrupt	=	Right Back Side	+	Abrupt	+	D
No	=	Right Back Side	+	No	+	D
Start	=	Right Back Side	+	Start	+	D
Father	=	Right Back Side	+	Father	+	D
Lose	=	Right Back Side	+	Lose	+	D
Absorb	=	Right Back Side	+	Absorb	+	D
Danger	=	Right Back Side	+	Danger	+	D
abate	=	Right Back Side	+	abate	+	D
Metre	=	Right Back Side	+	Metre	+	D
achieve	=	Right Back Side	+	achieve	+	D
Paper	=	Right Back Side	+	Paper	+	D
The	=	Right Back Side	+	The	+	D
As	=	Right Back Side	+	As	+	D
Tree of life	=	Left Back Side	+	Tree of life	+	D
Month	=	Right Back Side	+	Month	+	D
Is	=	Right Back Side	+	Is	+	D

Turn right	=	Right Back Side	+	Turn right	+ D
Rotate	=	Right Back Side	+	Rotate	+ D
Turn left	=	Right Back Side	+	Turn left	+ D
To	=	Right Back Side	+	To	+ D
Heaven	=	Left Back Side	+	Heaven	+ D
Observe	=	Right Back Side	+	Observe	+ D
How	=	Right Back Side	+	How	+ D
accountable	=	Right Back Side	+	accountable	+ D
Why	=	Right Back Side	+	Why	+ D
absence	=	Right Back Side	+	absence	+ D
accrue	=	Right Back Side	+	accrue	+ D
abundance	=	Right Back Side	+	abundance	+ D
able	=	Right Back Side	+	able	+ D
Fingers	=	Right Back Side	+	Fingers	+ D
abdomen	=	Right Back Side	+	abdomen	+ D
abolish	=	Right Back Side	+	abolish	+ D
acclaim	=	Right Back Side	+	acclaim	+ D
Ten	=	Right Front	+	Ten	+ D
Trinity	=	Left Back Side	+	Trinity	+ D

Safe	=	Right Back Side	+	Safe	+	D
God	=	Left Back Side	+	God	+	D
Bicycle	=	Right Back Side	+	Bicycle	+	D
Life	=	Left Back Side	+	Life	+	D
Second	=	Right Back Side	+	Second	+	D
whistle	=	Right Back Side	+	whistle	+	D
Government	=	Centre top head	+	Government	+	D
Death	=	Left Back Side	+	Death	+	D
First	=	Right Back Side	+	First	+	D
above	=	Right Back Side	+	above	+	D
accordance	=	Right Back Side	+	accordance	+	D
top	=	Right Back Side	+	top	+	D
Two hundred	=	Right Front	+	Two hundred	+	D
Three thousand	=	Left Front	+	Three thousand	+	D
They	=	Right Back Side	+	They	+	D
Tonight	=	Right Back Side	+	Tonight	+	D
Calendar.	=	Left Back Side	+	Calendar.	+	D
Holy spirit	=	Left Back Side	+	Holy spirit	+	D
Year	=	Right Back Side	+	Year	+	D
Spirit	=	Left Back Side	+	Spirit	+	D

One hundred	=	Right Front	+	One hundred	+	D
Always	=	Right Back Side	+	Always	+	D
Strict	=	Right Back Side	+	Strict	+	D
acquire	=	Right Back Side	+	acquire	+	D
acid	=	Right Back Side	+	acid	+	D
accuracy	=	Right Back Side	+	accuracy	+	D
accept	=	Right Back Side	+	accept	+	D
Subtract	=	Right Back Side	+	Subtract	+	D
Many	=	Right Back Side	+	Many	+	D
where	=	Right Back Side	+	where	+	D
Multiply	=	Right Back Side	+	Multiply	+	D
who	=	Right Back Side	+	who	+	D
How	=	Right Back Side	+	How	+	D
Judgement	=	Left Back Side	+	Judgement	+	D
Was	=	Right Back Side	+	Was	+	D
Box	=	Right Back Side	+	Box	+	D
apologise	=	Right Back Side	+	apologise	+	D
centre	=	Right Back Side	+	centre	+	D

cry	=	Right Back Side	+	cry	+	D
voice	=	Right Back Side	+	voice	+	D
Knickers	=	Left Back Side	+	Knickers	+	D
Trousers	=	Right Back Side	+	Trousers	+	D
a	=	Right Back Side	+	a	+	D
able	=	Right Back Side	+	able	+	D
about	=	Right Back Side	+	about	+	D
above	=	Right Back Side	+	above	+	D
act	=	Right Back Side	+	act	+	D
add	=	Right Back Side	+	add	+	D
afraid	=	Right Back Side	+	afraid	+	D
after	=	Right Back Side	+	after	+	D
again	=	Right Back Side	+	again	+	D
against	=	Right Back Side	+	against	+	D
age	=	Right Back Side	+	age	+	D
ago	=	Right Back Side	+	ago	+	D
agree	=	Right Back Side	+	agree	+	D
air	=	Right Back Side	+	air	+	D

all	=	Right Back Side	+	all	+	D
allow	=	Right Back Side	+	allow	+	D
also	=	Right Back Side	+	also	+	D
always	=	Right Back Side	+	always	+	D
among	=	Right Back Side	+	among	+	D
an	=	Right Back Side	+	an	+	D
and	=	Right Back Side	+	and	+	D
anger	=	Right Back Side	+	anger	+	D
animal	=	Right Back Side	+	animal	+	D
answer	=	Right Back Side	+	answer	+	D
any	=	Right Back Side	+	any	+	D
appear	=	Right Back Side	+	appear	+	D
apple	=	Right Back Side	+	apple	+	D
are	=	Right Back Side	+	are	+	D
area	=	Right Back Side	+	area	+	D
arm	=	Right Back Side	+	arm	+	D
arrange	=	Right Back Side	+	arrange	+	D
arrive	=	Right Back Side	+	arrive	+	D

art	=	Right Back Side	+	art	+	D
as	=	Right Back Side	+	as	+	D
ask	=	Right Back Side	+	ask	+	D
at	=	Right Back Side	+	at	+	D
atom	=	Right Back Side	+	atom	+	D
baby	=	Right Back Side	+	baby	+	D
bad	=	Right Back Side	+	bad	+	D
ball	=	Right Back Side	+	ball	+	D
band	=	Right Back Side	+	band	+	D
bank	=	Right Back Side	+	bank	+	D
bar	=	Right Back Side	+	bar	+	D
base	=	Right Back Side	+	base	+	D
basic	=	Right Back Side	+	basic	+	D
bat	=	Right Back Side	+	bat	+	D
be	=	Right Back Side	+	be	+	D
bear	=	Right Back Side	+	bear	+	D
beat	=	Right Back Side	+	beat	+	D
beauty	=	Right Back Side	+	beauty	+	D

bed	=	Right Back Side	+	bed	+	D
been	=	Right Back Side	+	been	+	D
before	=	Right Back Side	+	before	+	D
began	=	Right Back Side	+	began	+	D
begin	=	Right Back Side	+	begin	+	D
behind	=	Right Back Side	+	behind	+	D
bell	=	Right Back Side	+	bell	+	D
best	=	Right Back Side	+	best	+	D
better	=	Right Back Side	+	better	+	D
between	=	Right Back Side	+	between	+	D
big	=	Right Back Side	+	big	+	D
bird	=	Right Back Side	+	bird	+	D
bit	=	Right Back Side	+	bit	+	D
black	=	Right Back Side	+	black	+	D
block	=	Right Back Side	+	block	+	D
blood	=	Right Back Side	+	blood	+	D
blow	=	Right Back Side	+	blow	+	D
blue	=	Right Back Side	+	blue	+	D

board	=	Right Back Side	+	board	+	D
boat	=	Right Back Side	+	boat	+	D
body	=	Right Back Side	+	body	+	D
bone	=	Right Back Side	+	bone	+	D
book	=	Right Back Side	+	book	+	D
born	=	Right Back Side	+	born	+	D
both	=	Right Back Side	+	both	+	D
bought	=	Right Back Side	+	bought	+	D
box	=	Right Back Side	+	box	+	D
boy	=	Right Back Side	+	boy	+	D
branch	=	Right Back Side	+	branch	+	D
bread	=	Right Back Side	+	bread	+	D
break	=	Right Back Side	+	break	+	D
bright	=	Right Back Side	+	bright	+	D
bring	=	Right Back Side	+	bring	+	D
broad	=	Right Back Side	+	broad	+	D
broke	=	Right Back Side	+	broke	+	D
brother	=	Right Back Side	+	brother	+	D

brought	=	Right Back Side	+	brought	+ D
brown	=	Right Back Side	+	brown	+ D
build	=	Right Back Side	+	build	+ D
burn	=	Right Back Side	+	burn	+ D
busy	=	Right Back Side	+	busy	+ D
but	=	Right Back Side	+	but	+ D
buy	=	Right Back Side	+	buy	+ D
by	=	Right Back Side	+	by	+ D
call	=	Right Back Side	+	call	+ D
came	=	Right Back Side	+	came	+ D
camp	=	Right Back Side	+	camp	+ D
can	=	Right Back Side	+	can	+ D
capital	=	Right Back Side	+	capital	+ D
captain	=	Right Back Side	+	captain	+ D
car	=	Right Back Side	+	car	+ D
card	=	Right Back Side	+	card	+ D
care	=	Right Back Side	+	care	+ D
carry	=	Right Back Side	+	carry	+ D

case	=	Right Back Side	+	case	+	D
cat	=	Right Back Side	+	cat	+	D
catch	=	Right Back Side	+	catch	+	D
caught	=	Right Back Side	+	caught	+	D
cause	=	Right Back Side	+	cause	+	D
cell	=	Right Back Side	+	cell	+	D
cent	=	Right Back Side	+	cent	+	D
center	=	Right Back Side	+	center	+	D
century	=	Right Back Side	+	century	+	D
certain	=	Right Back Side	+	certain	+	D
chair	=	Right Back Side	+	chair	+	D
chance	=	Right Back Side	+	chance	+	D
change	=	Right Back Side	+	change	+	D
character	=	Right Back Side	+	character	+	D
charge	=	Right Back Side	+	charge	+	D
chart	=	Right Back Side	+	chart	+	D
check	=	Right Back Side	+	check	+	D
chick	=	Right Back Side	+	chick	+	D

chief	=	Right Back Side	+	chief	+	D
child	=	Right Back Side	+	child	+	D
children	=	Left Back Side	+	children	+	D
choose	=	Right Back Side	+	choose	+	D
chord	=	Right Back Side	+	chord	+	D
circle	=	Right Back Side	+	circle	+	D
city	=	Right Back Side	+	city	+	D
claim	=	Right Back Side	+	claim	+	D
class	=	Right Back Side	+	class	+	D
clean	=	Right Back Side	+	clean	+	D
clear	=	Right Back Side	+	clear	+	D
climb	=	Right Back Side	+	climb	+	D
clock	=	Right Back Side	+	clock	+	D
close	=	Right Back Side	+	close	+	D
clothe	=	Right Back Side	+	clothe	+	D
cloud	=	Right Back Side	+	cloud	+	D
coast	=	Right Back Side	+	coast	+	D
coat	=	Right Back Side	+	coat	+	D

cold	=	Right Back Side	+	cold	+	D
collect	=	Right Back Side	+	collect	+	D
colony	=	Right Back Side	+	colony	+	D
color	=	Right Back Side	+	color	+	D
column	=	Right Back Side	+	column	+	D
come	=	Right Back Side	+	come	+	D
common	=	Right Back Side	+	common	+	D
company	=	Right Back Side	+	company	+	D
compare	=	Right Back Side	+	compare	+	D
complete	=	Right Back Side	+	complete	+	D
condition	=	Right Back Side	+	condition	+	D
connect	=	Right Back Side	+	connect	+	D
consider	=	Right Back Side	+	consider	+	D
consonant	=	Right Back Side	+	consonant	+	D
contain	=	Right Back Side	+	contain	+	D
continent	=	Right Back Side	+	continent	+	D
continue	=	Right Back Side	+	continue	+	D
control	=	Right Back Side	+	control	+	D

cook	=	Right Back Side	+	cook	+ D
cool	=	Right Back Side	+	cool	+ D
copy	=	Right Back Side	+	copy	+ D
corn	=	Right Back Side	+	corn	+ D
corner	=	Right Back Side	+	corner	+ D
correct	=	Right Back Side	+	correct	+ D
cost	=	Right Back Side	+	cost	+ D
cotton	=	Right Back Side	+	cotton	+ D
could	=	Right Back Side	+	could	+ D
count	=	Right Back Side	+	count	+ D
country	=	Right Back Side	+	country	+ D
course	=	Right Back Side	+	course	+ D
cover	=	Right Back Side	+	cover	+ D
cow	=	Right Back Side	+	cow	+ D
crease	=	Right Back Side	+	crease	+ D
create	=	Right Back Side	+	create	+ D
crop	=	Right Back Side	+	crop	+ D
cross	=	Right Back Side	+	cross	+ D

crowd	=	Right Back Side	+	crowd	+	D
cry	=	Right Back Side	+	cry	+	D
current	=	Right Back Side	+	current	+	D
cut	=	Right Back Side	+	cut	+	D
dad	=	Right Back Side	+	dad	+	D
dance	=	Right Back Side	+	dance	+	D
danger	=	Right Back Side	+	danger	+	D
dark	=	Right Back Side	+	dark	+	D
day	=	Right Back Side	+	day	+	D
dead	=	Left Back Side	+	dead	+	D
deal	=	Right Back Side	+	deal	+	D
dear	=	Right Back Side	+	dear	+	D
death	=	Right Back Side	+	death	+	D
decide	=	Right Back Side	+	decide	+	D
decimal	=	Right Back Side	+	decimal	+	D
deep	=	Right Back Side	+	deep	+	D
degree	=	Right Back Side	+	degree	+	D
depend on	=	Right Back Side	+	depend on	+	D

describe	=	Right Back Side	+	describe	+	D
desert	=	Right Back Side	+	desert	+	D
design	=	Right Back Side	+	design	+	D
determine	=	Right Back Side	+	determine	+	D
develop	=	Right Back Side	+	develop	+	D
dictionary	=	Right Back Side	+	dictionary	+	D
did	=	Right Back Side	+	did	+	D
die	=	Right Back Side	+	die	+	D
differ	=	Right Back Side	+	differ	+	D
difficult	=	Right Back Side	+	difficult	+	D
direct	=	Right Back Side	+	direct	+	D
discuss	=	Right Back Side	+	discuss	+	D
distant	=	Right Back Side	+	distant	+	D
divide	=	Right Back Side	+	divide	+	D
division	=	Right Back Side	+	division	+	D
doctor	=	Right Back Side	+	doctor	+	D
does	=	Right Back Side	+	does	+	D
dog	=	Right Back Side	+	dog	+	D

dollar	=	Right Back Side	+	dollar	+	D
done	=	Right Back Side	+	done	+	D
do not	=	Right Back Side	+	do not	+	D
door	=	Right Back Side	+	door	+	D
double	=	Right Back Side	+	double	+	D
draw	=	Right Back Side	+	draw	+	D
dream	=	Right Back Side	+	dream	+	D
dress	=	Left Back Side	+	dress	+	D
drink	=	Right Back Side	+	drink	+	D
drive	=	Right Back Side	+	drive	+	D
drop	=	Right Back Side	+	drop	+	D
dry	=	Right Back Side	+	dry	+	D
duck	=	Right Back Side	+	duck	+	D
during	=	Right Back Side	+	during	+	D
each	=	Right Back Side	+	each	+	D
ear	=	Right Back Side	+	ear	+	D
early	=	Right Back Side	+	early	+	D
earth	=	Right Back Side	+	earth	+	D

ease	=	Right Back Side	+	ease	+	D
east	=	Right Back Side	+	east	+	D
eat	=	Right Back Side	+	eat	+	D
edge	=	Right Back Side	+	edge	+	D
effect	=	Right Back Side	+	effect	+	D
egg	=	Right Back Side	+	egg	+	D
eight	=	Right Back Side	+	eight	+	D
either	=	Right Back Side	+	either	+	D
electric	=	Right Back Side	+	electric	+	D
element	=	Right Back Side	+	element	+	D
else	=	Right Back Side	+	else	+	D
enemy	=	Right Back Side	+	enemy	+	D
energy	=	Right Back Side	+	energy	+	D
engine	=	Right Back Side	+	engine	+	D
enough	=	Right Back Side	+	enough	+	D
enter	=	Right Back Side	+	enter	+	D
equal	=	Right Back Side	+	equal	+	D
equate	=	Right Back Side	+	equate	+	D

especially	=	Right Back Side	+	especially	+ D
even	=	Right Back Side	+	even	+ D
evening	=	Right Back Side	+	evening	+ D
event	=	Right Back Side	+	event	+ D
ever	=	Right Back Side	+	ever	+ D
every	=	Right Back Side	+	every	+ D
exact	=	Right Back Side	+	exact	+ D
example	=	Right Back Side	+	example	+ D
except	=	Right Back Side	+	except	+ D
excite	=	Right Back Side	+	excite	+ D
exercise	=	Right Back Side	+	exercise	+ D
exhale	=	Right Back Side	+	exhale	+ D
expect	=	Right Back Side	+	expect	+ D
experience	=	Right Back Side	+	experience	+ D
experiment	=	Right Back Side	+	experiment	+ D
eye	=	Right Back Side	+	eye	+ D
face	=	Right Back Side	+	face	+ D
fact	=	Right Back Side	+	fact	+ D

fair	=	Right Back Side	+	fair	+	D
fall	=	Right Back Side	+	fall	+	D
family	=	Right Back Side	+	family	+	D
famous	=	Right Back Side	+	famous	+	D
far	=	Right Back Side	+	far	+	D
farm	=	Right Back Side	+	farm	+	D
fast	=	Right Back Side	+	fast	+	D
fat	=	Right Back Side	+	fat	+	D
favor	=	Right Back Side	+	favor	+	D
fear	=	Right Back Side	+	fear	+	D
feed	=	Right Back Side	+	feed	+	D
feel	=	Right Back Side	+	feel	+	D
feet	=	Right Back Side	+	feet	+	D
fell	=	Right Back Side	+	fell	+	D
felt	=	Right Back Side	+	felt	+	D
few	=	Right Back Side	+	few	+	D
field	=	Right Back Side	+	field	+	D
fig	=	Right Back Side	+	fig	+	D

fight	=	Right Back Side	+	fight	+	D
figure	=	Right Back Side	+	figure	+	D
fill	=	Right Back Side	+	fill	+	D
final	=	Right Back Side	+	final	+	D
find	=	Right Back Side	+	find	+	D
fine	=	Right Back Side	+	fine	+	D
finger	=	Right Back Side	+	finger	+	D
finish	=	Right Back Side	+	finish	+	D
fire	=	Right Back Side	+	fire	+	D
first	=	Right Back Side	+	first	+	D
fish	=	Right Back Side	+	fish	+	D
fit	=	Right Back Side	+	fit	+	D
five	=	Right Back Side	+	five	+	D
flat	=	Right Back Side	+	flat	+	D
floor	=	Right Back Side	+	floor	+	D
flow	=	Right Back Side	+	flow	+	D
flower	=	Right Back Side	+	flower	+	D
fly	=	Right Back Side	+	fly	+	D

follow	=	Right Back Side	+	follow	+	D
food	=	Right Back Side	+	food	+	D
foot	=	Right Back Side	+	foot	+	D
for	=	Right Back Side	+	for	+	D
force	=	Right Back Side	+	force	+	D
forest	=	Right Back Side	+	forest	+	D
form	=	Right Back Side	+	form	+	D
forward	=	Right Back Side	+	forward	+	D
found	=	Right Back Side	+	found	+	D
four	=	Right Back Side	+	four	+	D
fraction	=	Right Back Side	+	fraction	+	D
free	=	Right Back Side	+	free	+	D
fresh	=	Right Back Side	+	fresh	+	D
friend	=	Right Back Side	+	friend	+	D
from	=	Right Back Side	+	from	+	D
fruit	=	Right Back Side	+	fruit	+	D
full	=	Right Back Side	+	full	+	D
fun	=	Right Back Side	+	fun	+	D

game	=	Right Back Side	+	game	+ D
garden	=	Right Back Side	+	garden	+ D
gas	=	Right Back Side	+	gas	+ D
gather	=	Right Back Side	+	gather	+ D
gave	=	Right Back Side	+	gave	+ D
general	=	Right Back Side	+	general	+ D
gentle	=	Right Back Side	+	gentle	+ D
get	=	Right Back Side	+	get	+ D
girl	=	Left Back Side	+	girl	+ D
give	=	Right Back Side	+	give	+ D
glad	=	Right Back Side	+	glad	+ D
glass	=	Right Back Side	+	glass	+ D
go	=	Right Back Side	+	go	+ D
gold	=	Right Back Side	+	gold	+ D
gone	=	Right Back Side	+	gone	+ D
good	=	Right Back Side	+	good	+ D
got	=	Right Back Side	+	got	+ D
govern	=	Right Back Side	+	govern	+ D

grand	=	Right Back Side	+	grand	+	D
grass	=	Right Back Side	+	grass	+	D
Gray	=	Right Back Side	+	Gray	+	D
great	=	Right Back Side	+	great	+	D
green	=	Right Back Side	+	green	+	D
grew	=	Right Back Side	+	grew	+	D
ground	=	Right Back Side	+	ground	+	D
group	=	Right Back Side	+	group	+	D
grow	=	Right Back Side	+	grow	+	D
guess	=	Right Back Side	+	guess	+	D
guide	=	Right Back Side	+	guide	+	D
gun	=	Right Back Side	+	gun	+	D
had	=	Right Back Side	+	had	+	D
hair	=	Right Back Side	+	hair	+	D
half	=	Right Back Side	+	half	+	D
hand	=	Right Back Side	+	hand	+	D
happen	=	Right Back Side	+	happen	+	D
happy	=	Right Back Side	+	happy	+	D

hard	=	Right Back Side	+	hard	+	D
has	=	Right Back Side	+	has	+	D
hat	=	Right Back Side	+	hat	+	D
have	=	Right Back Side	+	have	+	D
he	=	Right Back Side	+	he	+	D
head	=	Right Back Side	+	head	+	D
hear	=	Right Back Side	+	hear	+	D
heard	=	Right Back Side	+	heard	+	D
heart	=	Right Back Side	+	heart	+	D
heat	=	Right Back Side	+	heat	+	D
heavy	=	Right Back Side	+	heavy	+	D
held	=	Right Back Side	+	held	+	D
help	=	Right Back Side	+	help	+	D
her	=	Left Back Side	+	her	+	D
here	=	Right Back Side	+	here	+	D
hill	=	Right Back Side	+	hill	+	D
him	=	Right Back Side	+	him	+	D
his	=	Right Back Side	+	his	+	D

history	=	Right Back Side	+	history	+	D
hit	=	Right Back Side	+	hit	+	D
hold	=	Right Back Side	+	hold	+	D
hole	=	Right Back Side	+	hole	+	D
home	=	Right Back Side	+	home	+	D
hope	=	Right Back Side	+	hope	+	D
horse	=	Right Back Side	+	horse	+	D
hot	=	Right Back Side	+	hot	+	D
hour	=	Right Back Side	+	hour	+	D
house	=	Right Back Side	+	house	+	D
how	=	Right Back Side	+	how	+	D
huge	=	Right Back Side	+	huge	+	D
human	=	Right Back Side	+	human	+	D
hundred	=	Right Back Side	+	hundred	+	D
hunt	=	Right Back Side	+	hunt	+	D
hurry	=	Right Back Side	+	hurry	+	D
I	=	Right Back Side	+	I	+	D
ice	=	Right Back Side	+	ice	+	D

idea	=	Right Back Side	+	idea	+	D
if	=	Right Back Side	+	if	+	D
imagine	=	Right Back Side	+	imagine	+	D
in	=	Right Back Side	+	in	+	D
inch	=	Right Back Side	+	inch	+	D
include	=	Right Back Side	+	include	+	D
indicate	=	Right Back Side	+	indicate	+	D
industry	=	Right Back Side	+	industry	+	D
insect	=	Right Back Side	+	insect	+	D
instant	=	Right Back Side	+	instant	+	D
instrument	=	Right Back Side	+	instrument	+	D
interest	=	Right Back Side	+	interest	+	D
invent	=	Right Back Side	+	invent	+	D
iron	=	Right Back Side	+	iron	+	D
is	=	Right Back Side	+	is	+	D
island	=	Right Back Side	+	island	+	D
it	=	Right Back Side	+	it	+	D
job	=	Right Back Side	+	job	+	D

join	=	Right Back Side	+	join	+	D
joy	=	Right Back Side	+	joy	+	D
jump	=	Right Back Side	+	jump	+	D
just	=	Right Back Side	+	just	+	D
keep	=	Right Back Side	+	keep	+	D
kept	=	Right Back Side	+	kept	+	D
key	=	Right Back Side	+	key	+	D
kill	=	Right Back Side	+	kill	+	D
kind	=	Right Back Side	+	kind	+	D
king	=	Right Back Side	+	king	+	D
knew	=	Right Back Side	+	knew	+	D
know	=	Right Back Side	+	know	+	D
lady	=	Right Back Side	+	lady	+	D
lake	=	Right Back Side	+	lake	+	D
land	=	Right Back Side	+	land	+	D
language	=	Right Back Side	+	language	+	D
large	=	Right Back Side	+	large	+	D
last	=	Right Back Side	+	last	+	D

late	=	Right Back Side	+	late	+	D
laugh	=	Right Back Side	+	laugh	+	D
law	=	Right Back Side	+	law	+	D
lay	=	Right Back Side	+	lay	+	D
lead	=	Right Back Side	+	lead	+	D
learn	=	Right Back Side	+	learn	+	D
least	=	Right Back Side	+	least	+	D
leave	=	Right Back Side	+	leave	+	D
led	=	Right Back Side	+	led	+	D
left	=	Right Back Side	+	left	+	D
length	=	Right Back Side	+	length	+	D
less	=	Right Back Side	+	less	+	D
let	=	Right Back Side	+	let	+	D
letter	=	Right Back Side	+	letter	+	D
level	=	Right Back Side	+	level	+	D
lie	=	Right Back Side	+	lie	+	D
life	=	Right Back Side	+	life	+	D
lift	=	Right Back Side	+	lift	+	D

light	=	Right Back Side	+	light	+ D
like	=	Right Back Side	+	like	+ D
line	=	Right Back Side	+	line	+ D
liquid	=	Right Back Side	+	liquid	+ D
list	=	Right Back Side	+	list	+ D
listen	=	Right Back Side	+	listen	+ D
little	=	Right Back Side	+	little	+ D
live	=	Right Back Side	+	live	+ D
locate	=	Right Back Side	+	locate	+ D
log	=	Right Back Side	+	log	+ D
lone	=	Right Back Side	+	lone	+ D
long	=	Right Back Side	+	long	+ D
look	=	Right Back Side	+	look	+ D
lost	=	Right Back Side	+	lost	+ D
lot	=	Right Back Side	+	lot	+ D
loud	=	Right Back Side	+	loud	+ D
love	=	Right Back Side	+	love	+ D
low	=	Right Back Side	+	low	+ D

machine	=	Right Back Side	+	machine	+	D
made	=	Right Back Side	+	made	+	D
magnet	=	Right Back Side	+	magnet	+	D
main	=	Right Back Side	+	main	+	D
major	=	Right Back Side	+	major	+	D
make	=	Right Back Side	+	make	+	D
many	=	Right Back Side	+	many	+	D
map	=	Right Back Side	+	map	+	D
mark	=	Right Back Side	+	mark	+	D
market	=	Right Back Side	+	market	+	D
mass	=	Right Back Side	+	mass	+	D
master	=	Right Back Side	+	master	+	D
match	=	Right Back Side	+	match	+	D
material	=	Right Back Side	+	material	+	D
matter	=	Right Back Side	+	matter	+	D
may	=	Right Back Side	+	may	+	D
me	=	Right Back Side	+	me	+	D
mean	=	Right Back Side	+	mean	+	D

meant	=	Right Back Side	+	meant	+	D
measure	=	Right Back Side	+	measure	+	D
meat	=	Right Back Side	+	meat	+	D
meet	=	Right Back Side	+	meet	+	D
melody	=	Right Back Side	+	melody	+	D
men	=	Right Back Side	+	men	+	D
metal	=	Right Back Side	+	metal	+	D
method	=	Right Back Side	+	method	+	D
might	=	Right Back Side	+	might	+	D
mile	=	Right Back Side	+	mile	+	D
milk	=	Right Back Side	+	milk	+	D
million	=	Right Back Side	+	million	+	D
mind	=	Right Back Side	+	mind	+	D
mine	=	Right Back Side	+	mine	+	D
minute	=	Right Back Side	+	minute	+	D
miss	=	Right Back Side	+	miss	+	D
mix	=	Right Back Side	+	mix	+	D
modern	=	Right Back Side	+	modern	+	D

molecule	=	Right Back Side	+	molecule	+ D
moment	=	Right Back Side	+	moment	+ D
money	=	Right Back Side	+	money	+ D
month	=	Right Back Side	+	month	+ D
moon	=	Right Back Side	+	moon	+ D
more	=	Right Back Side	+	more	+ D
morning	=	Right Back Side	+	morning	+ D
most	=	Right Back Side	+	most	+ D
mother	=	Left Back Side	+	mother	+ D
motion	=	Right Back Side	+	motion	+ D
mount	=	Right Back Side	+	mount	+ D
mountain	=	Right Back Side	+	mountain	+ D
mouth	=	Right Back Side	+	mouth	+ D
move	=	Right Back Side	+	move	+ D
much	=	Right Back Side	+	much	+ D
multiply	=	Right Back Side	+	multiply	+ D
music	=	Right Back Side	+	music	+ D
must	=	Right Back Side	+	must	+ D

my	=	Right Back Side	+	my	+	D
name	=	Right Back Side	+	name	+	D
nation	=	Right Back Side	+	nation	+	D
natural	=	Right Back Side	+	natural	+	D
nature	=	Right Back Side	+	nature	+	D
near	=	Right Back Side	+	near	+	D
necessary	=	Right Back Side	+	necessary	+	D
neck	=	Right Back Side	+	neck	+	D
need	=	Right Back Side	+	need	+	D
neighbors	=	Right Back Side	+	neighbors	+	D
never	=	Right Back Side	+	never	+	D
new	=	Right Back Side	+	new	+	D
next	=	Right Back Side	+	next	+	D
night	=	Right Back Side	+	night	+	D
nine	=	Right Back Side	+	nine	+	D
no	=	Right Back Side	+	no	+	D
noise	=	Right Back Side	+	noise	+	D
noon	=	Right Back Side	+	noon	+	D

nor	=	Right Back Side	+	nor	+	D
north	=	Right Back Side	+	north	+	D
nose	=	Right Back Side	+	nose	+	D
not	=	Right Back Side	+	not	+	D
note	=	Right Back Side	+	note	+	D
nothing	=	Right Back Side	+	nothing	+	D
notice	=	Right Back Side	+	notice	+	D
noun	=	Right Back Side	+	noun	+	D
now	=	Right Back Side	+	now	+	D
number	=	Right Back Side	+	number	+	D
numeral	=	Right Back Side	+	numeral	+	D
object	=	Right Back Side	+	object	+	D
observe	=	Right Back Side	+	observe	+	D
occur	=	Right Back Side	+	occur	+	D
ocean	=	Right Back Side	+	ocean	+	D
of	=	Right Back Side	+	of	+	D
off	=	Right Back Side	+	off	+	D
offer	=	Right Back Side	+	offer	+	D

office	=	Right Back Side	+	office	+	D
often	=	Right Back Side	+	often	+	D
oh	=	Right Back Side	+	oh	+	D
oil	=	Right Back Side	+	oil	+	D
old	=	Right Back Side	+	old	+	D
on	=	Right Back Side	+	on	+	D
once	=	Right Back Side	+	once	+	D
one	=	Right Back Side	+	one	+	D
only	=	Right Back Side	+	only	+	D
open	=	Right Back Side	+	open	+	D
operate	=	Right Back Side	+	operate	+	D
opposite	=	Right Back Side	+	opposite	+	D
order	=	Right Back Side	+	order	+	D
organ	=	Right Back Side	+	organ	+	D
original	=	Right Back Side	+	original	+	D
other	=	Right Back Side	+	other	+	D
our	=	Right Back Side	+	our	+	D
out	=	Right Back Side	+	out	+	D

over	=	Right Back Side	+	over	+	D
own	=	Right Back Side	+	own	+	D
oxygen	=	Right Back Side	+	oxygen	+	D
page	=	Right Back Side	+	page	+	D
paint	=	Right Back Side	+	paint	+	D
pair	=	Right Back Side	+	pair	+	D
paper	=	Right Back Side	+	paper	+	D
paragraph	=	Right Back Side	+	paragraph	+	D
parent	=	Right Back Side	+	parent	+	D
part	=	Right Back Side	+	part	+	D
particular	=	Right Back Side	+	particular	+	D
party	=	Right Back Side	+	party	+	D
pass	=	Right Back Side	+	pass	+	D
past	=	Right Back Side	+	past	+	D
path	=	Right Back Side	+	path	+	D
pattern	=	Right Back Side	+	pattern	+	D
pay	=	Right Back Side	+	pay	+	D
people	=	Right Back Side	+	people	+	D

perhaps	=	Right Back Side	+	perhaps	+	D
period	=	Right Back Side	+	period	+	D
person	=	Right Back Side	+	person	+	D
phrase	=	Right Back Side	+	phrase	+	D
pick	=	Right Back Side	+	pick	+	D
picture	=	Right Back Side	+	picture	+	D
piece	=	Right Back Side	+	piece	+	D
pitch	=	Right Back Side	+	pitch	+	D
place	=	Right Back Side	+	place	+	D
plain	=	Right Back Side	+	plain	+	D
plan	=	Right Back Side	+	plan	+	D
plane	=	Right Back Side	+	plane	+	D
planet	=	Right Back Side	+	planet	+	D
plant	=	Right Back Side	+	plant	+	D
play	=	Right Back Side	+	play	+	D
please	=	Right Back Side	+	please	+	D
plural	=	Right Back Side	+	plural	+	D
poem	=	Right Back Side	+	poem	+	D

point	=	Right Back Side	+	point	+	D
poor	=	Right Back Side	+	poor	+	D
populate	=	Right Back Side	+	populate	+	D
port	=	Right Back Side	+	port	+	D
pose	=	Right Back Side	+	pose	+	D
position	=	Right Back Side	+	position	+	D
possible	=	Right Back Side	+	possible	+	D
post	=	Right Back Side	+	post	+	D
pound	=	Right Back Side	+	pound	+	D
power	=	Right Back Side	+	power	+	D
practice	=	Right Back Side	+	practice	+	D
prepare	=	Right Back Side	+	prepare	+	D
present	=	Right Back Side	+	present	+	D
press	=	Right Back Side	+	press	+	D
pretty	=	Right Back Side	+	pretty	+	D
print	=	Right Back Side	+	print	+	D
probable	=	Right Back Side	+	probable	+	D
problem	=	Right Back Side	+	problem	+	D

process	=	Right Back Side	+	process	+	D
produce	=	Right Back Side	+	produce	+	D
product	=	Right Back Side	+	product	+	D
proper	=	Right Back Side	+	proper	+	D
property	=	Right Back Side	+	property	+	D
protect	=	Right Back Side	+	protect	+	D
prove	=	Right Back Side	+	prove	+	D
provide	=	Right Back Side	+	provide	+	D
pull	=	Right Back Side	+	pull	+	D
push	=	Right Back Side	+	push	+	D
put	=	Right Back Side	+	put	+	D
quart	=	Right Back Side	+	quart	+	D
question	=	Right Back Side	+	question	+	D
quick	=	Right Back Side	+	quick	+	D
quiet	=	Right Back Side	+	quiet	+	D
quite	=	Right Back Side	+	quite	+	D
quotient	=	Right Back Side	+	quotient	+	D
race	=	Right Back Side	+	race	+	D

radio	=	Right Back Side	+	radio	+	D
rail	=	Right Back Side	+	rail	+	D
rain	=	Right Back Side	+	rain	+	D
raise	=	Right Back Side	+	raise	+	D
ran	=	Right Back Side	+	ran	+	D
range	=	Right Back Side	+	range	+	D
rather	=	Right Back Side	+	rather	+	D
reach	=	Right Back Side	+	reach	+	D
read	=	Right Back Side	+	read	+	D
ready	=	Right Back Side	+	ready	+	D
real	=	Right Back Side	+	real	+	D
reason	=	Right Back Side	+	reason	+	D
receive	=	Right Back Side	+	receive	+	D
record	=	Right Back Side	+	record	+	D
red	=	Right Back Side	+	red	+	D
region	=	Right Back Side	+	region	+	D
remember	=	Right Back Side	+	remember	+	D
repeat	=	Right Back Side	+	repeat	+	D

reply	=	Right Back Side	+	reply	+	D
represent	=	Right Back Side	+	represent	+	D
require	=	Right Back Side	+	require	+	D
rest	=	Right Back Side	+	rest	+	D
result	=	Right Back Side	+	result	+	D
rich	=	Right Back Side	+	rich	+	D
ride	=	Right Back Side	+	ride	+	D
right	=	Right Back Side	+	right	+	D
ring	=	Right Back Side	+	ring	+	D
rise	=	Right Back Side	+	rise	+	D
river	=	Right Back Side	+	river	+	D
road	=	Right Back Side	+	road	+	D
rock	=	Right Back Side	+	rock	+	D
roll	=	Right Back Side	+	roll	+	D
room	=	Right Back Side	+	room	+	D
root	=	Right Back Side	+	root	+	D
rope	=	Right Back Side	+	rope	+	D
rose	=	Right Back Side	+	rose	+	D

round	=	Right Back Side	+	round	+	D
row	=	Right Back Side	+	row	+	D
rub	=	Right Back Side	+	rub	+	D
rule	=	Right Back Side	+	rule	+	D
safe	=	Right Back Side	+	safe	+	D
said	=	Right Back Side	+	said	+	D
sail	=	Right Back Side	+	sail	+	D
salt	=	Right Back Side	+	salt	+	D
same	=	Right Back Side	+	same	+	D
sand	=	Right Back Side	+	sand	+	D
sat	=	Right Back Side	+	sat	+	D
save	=	Right Back Side	+	save	+	D
saw	=	Right Back Side	+	saw	+	D
say	=	Right Back Side	+	say	+	D
scale	=	Right Back Side	+	scale	+	D
school	=	Right Back Side	+	school	+	D
science	=	Right Back Side	+	science	+	D
score	=	Right Back Side	+	score	+	D

sea	=	Right Back Side	+	sea	+	D
search	=	Right Back Side	+	search	+	D
season	=	Right Back Side	+	season	+	D
seat	=	Right Back Side	+	seat	+	D
second	=	Right Back Side	+	second	+	D
section	=	Right Back Side	+	section	+	D
see	=	Right Back Side	+	see	+	D
seed	=	Right Back Side	+	seed	+	D
seem	=	Right Back Side	+	seem	+	D
segment	=	Right Back Side	+	segment	+	D
select	=	Right Back Side	+	select	+	D
self	=	Right Back Side	+	self	+	D
sell	=	Right Back Side	+	sell	+	D
send	=	Right Back Side	+	send	+	D
sense	=	Right Back Side	+	sense	+	D
sent	=	Right Back Side	+	sent	+	D
sentence	=	Right Back Side	+	sentence	+	D
separate	=	Right Back Side	+	separate	+	D

serve	=	Right Back Side	+	serve	+	D
set	=	Right Back Side	+	set	+	D
settle	=	Right Back Side	+	settle	+	D
seven	=	Right Back Side	+	seven	+	D
several	=	Right Back Side	+	several	+	D
shall	=	Right Back Side	+	shall	+	D
shape	=	Right Back Side	+	shape	+	D
share	=	Right Back Side	+	share	+	D
sharp	=	Right Back Side	+	sharp	+	D
she	=	Left Back Side	+	she	+	D
sheet	=	Right Back Side	+	sheet	+	D
shell	=	Right Back Side	+	shell	+	D
shine	=	Right Back Side	+	shine	+	D
ship	=	Right Back Side	+	ship	+	D
shoe	=	Right Back Side	+	shoe	+	D
shop	=	Right Back Side	+	shop	+	D
shore	=	Right Back Side	+	shore	+	D
short	=	Right Back Side	+	short	+	D

should	=	Right Back Side	+	should	+	D
shoulder	=	Right Back Side	+	shoulder	+	D
shout	=	Right Back Side	+	shout	+	D
show	=	Right Back Side	+	show	+	D
side	=	Right Back Side	+	side	+	D
sight	=	Right Back Side	+	sight	+	D
sign	=	Right Back Side	+	sign	+	D
silent	=	Right Back Side	+	silent	+	D
silver	=	Right Back Side	+	silver	+	D
similar	=	Right Back Side	+	similar	+	D
simple	=	Right Back Side	+	simple	+	D
since	=	Right Back Side	+	since	+	D
single	=	Right Back Side	+	single	+	D
sister	=	Right Back Side	+	sister	+	D
six	=	Right Back Side	+	six	+	D
size	=	Right Back Side	+	size	+	D
skill	=	Right Back Side	+	skill	+	D
skin	=	Right Back Side	+	skin	+	D

sky	=	Right Back Side	+	sky	+	D
slave	=	Right Back Side	+	slave	+	D
sleep	=	Right Back Side	+	sleep	+	D
slip	=	Right Back Side	+	slip	+	D
slow	=	Right Back Side	+	slow	+	D
small	=	Right Back Side	+	small	+	D
smell	=	Right Back Side	+	smell	+	D
smile	=	Right Back Side	+	smile	+	D
snow	=	Right Back Side	+	snow	+	D
so	=	Right Back Side	+	so	+	D
soft	=	Right Back Side	+	soft	+	D
soil	=	Right Back Side	+	soil	+	D
soldier	=	Right Back Side	+	soldier	+	D
solution	=	Right Back Side	+	solution	+	D
solve	=	Right Back Side	+	solve	+	D
some	=	Right Back Side	+	some	+	D
son	=	Right Back Side	+	son	+	D
song	=	Right Back Side	+	song	+	D

soon	=	Right Back Side	+	soon	+	D
sound	=	Right Back Side	+	sound	+	D
south	=	Right Back Side	+	south	+	D
space	=	Right Back Side	+	space	+	D
speak	=	Right Back Side	+	speak	+	D
special	=	Right Back Side	+	special	+	D
speech	=	Right Back Side	+	speech	+	D
speed	=	Right Back Side	+	speed	+	D
spell	=	Right Back Side	+	spell	+	D
spend	=	Right Back Side	+	spend	+	D
spoke	=	Right Back Side	+	spoke	+	D
spot	=	Right Back Side	+	spot	+	D
spread	=	Right Back Side	+	spread	+	D
spring	=	Right Back Side	+	spring	+	D
square	=	Right Back Side	+	square	+	D
stand	=	Right Back Side	+	stand	+	D
star	=	Right Back Side	+	star	+	D
start	=	Right Back Side	+	start	+	D

state	=	Right Back Side	+	state	+	D
station	=	Right Back Side	+	station	+	D
stay	=	Right Back Side	+	stay	+	D
stead	=	Right Back Side	+	stead	+	D
steam	=	Right Back Side	+	steam	+	D
steel	=	Right Back Side	+	steel	+	D
step	=	Right Back Side	+	step	+	D
stick	=	Right Back Side	+	stick	+	D
still	=	Right Back Side	+	still	+	D
stone	=	Right Back Side	+	stone	+	D
stood	=	Right Back Side	+	stood	+	D
stop	=	Right Back Side	+	stop	+	D
store	=	Right Back Side	+	store	+	D
story	=	Right Back Side	+	story	+	D
straight	=	Right Back Side	+	straight	+	D
strange	=	Right Back Side	+	strange	+	D
stream	=	Right Back Side	+	stream	+	D
street	=	Right Back Side	+	street	+	D

stretch	=	Right Back Side	+	stretch	+	D
string	=	Right Back Side	+	string	+	D
strong	=	Right Back Side	+	strong	+	D
student	=	Right Back Side	+	student	+	D
study	=	Right Back Side	+	study	+	D
subject	=	Right Back Side	+	subject	+	D
substance	=	Right Back Side	+	substance	+	D
subtract	=	Right Back Side	+	subtract	+	D
success	=	Right Back Side	+	success	+	D
such	=	Right Back Side	+	such	+	D
sudden	=	Right Back Side	+	sudden	+	D
suffix	=	Right Back Side	+	suffix	+	D
sugar	=	Right Back Side	+	sugar	+	D
suggest	=	Right Back Side	+	suggest	+	D
suit	=	Right Back Side	+	suit	+	D
summer	=	Right Back Side	+	summer	+	D
sun	=	Right Back Side	+	sun	+	D
supply	=	Right Back Side	+	supply	+	D

support	=	Right Back Side	+	support	+	D
sure	=	Right Back Side	+	sure	+	D
surface	=	Right Back Side	+	surface	+	D
surprise	=	Right Back Side	+	surprise	+	D
swim	=	Right Back Side	+	swim	+	D
syllable	=	Right Back Side	+	syllable	+	D
symbol	=	Right Back Side	+	symbol	+	D
system	=	Right Back Side	+	system	+	D
table	=	Right Back Side	+	table	+	D
tail	=	Right Back Side	+	tail	+	D
take	=	Right Back Side	+	take	+	D
tall	=	Right Back Side	+	tall	+	D
teach	=	Right Back Side	+	teach	+	D
team	=	Right Back Side	+	team	+	D
teeth	=	Right Back Side	+	teeth	+	D
tell	=	Right Back Side	+	tell	+	D
temperature	=	Right Back Side	+	temperature	+	D
ten	=	Right Back Side	+	ten	+	D

term	=	Right Back Side	+	term	+	D
than	=	Right Back Side	+	than	+	D
thank	=	Right Back Side	+	thank	+	D
that	=	Right Back Side	+	that	+	D
their	=	Right Back Side	+	their	+	D
them	=	Right Back Side	+	them	+	D
then	=	Right Back Side	+	then	+	D
there	=	Right Back Side	+	there	+	D
these	=	Right Back Side	+	these	+	D
they	=	Right Back Side	+	they	+	D
thick	=	Right Back Side	+	thick	+	D
thin	=	Right Back Side	+	thin	+	D
thing	=	Right Back Side	+	thing	+	D
think	=	Right Back Side	+	think	+	D
third	=	Right Back Side	+	third	+	D
those	=	Right Back Side	+	those	+	D
though	=	Right Back Side	+	though	+	D
thought	=	Right Back Side	+	thought	+	D

thousand	=	Right Front	+	thousand	+	D
three	=	Right Back Side	+	three	+	D
through	=	Right Back Side	+	through	+	D
throw	=	Right Back Side	+	throw	+	D
thus	=	Right Back Side	+	thus	+	D
tie	=	Right Back Side	+	tie	+	D
time	=	Right Back Side	+	time	+	D
tiny	=	Right Back Side	+	tiny	+	D
tire	=	Right Back Side	+	tire	+	D
to	=	Right Back Side	+	to	+	D
together	=	Right Back Side	+	together	+	D
told	=	Right Back Side	+	told	+	D
tone	=	Right Back Side	+	tone	+	D
too	=	Right Back Side	+	too	+	D
took	=	Right Back Side	+	took	+	D
tool	=	Right Back Side	+	tool	+	D
total	=	Right Back Side	+	total	+	D
toward	=	Right Back Side	+	toward	+	D

town	=	Right Back Side	+	town	+ D
track	=	Right Back Side	+	track	+ D
trade	=	Right Back Side	+	trade	+ D
train	=	Right Back Side	+	train	+ D
travel	=	Right Back Side	+	travel	+ D
tree	=	Right Back Side	+	tree	+ D
triangle	=	Right Back Side	+	triangle	+ D
trip	=	Right Back Side	+	trip	+ D
trouble	=	Right Back Side	+	trouble	+ D
truck	=	Right Back Side	+	truck	+ D
try	=	Right Back Side	+	try	+ D
tube	=	Right Back Side	+	tube	+ D
turn	=	Right Back Side	+	turn	+ D
twenty	=	Right Back Side	+	twenty	+ D
two	=	Right Back Side	+	two	+ D
type	=	Right Back Side	+	type	+ D
under	=	Right Back Side	+	under	+ D
unit	=	Right Back Side	+	unit	+ D

until	=	Right Back Side	+	until	+	D
us	=	Right Back Side	+	us	+	D
use	=	Right Back Side	+	use	+	D
usual	=	Right Back Side	+	usual	+	D
valley	=	Right Back Side	+	valley	+	D
value	=	Right Back Side	+	value	+	D
vary	=	Right Back Side	+	vary	+	D
verb	=	Right Back Side	+	verb	+	D
very	=	Right Back Side	+	very	+	D
view	=	Right Back Side	+	view	+	D
village	=	Right Back Side	+	village	+	D
visit	=	Right Back Side	+	visit	+	D
vowel	=	Right Back Side	+	vowel	+	D
wait	=	Right Back Side	+	wait	+	D
walk	=	Right Back Side	+	walk	+	D
wall	=	Right Back Side	+	wall	+	D
want	=	Right Back Side	+	want	+	D
war	=	Right Back Side	+	war	+	D

warm	=	Right Back Side	+	warm	+	D
wash	=	Right Back Side	+	wash	+	D
watch	=	Right Back Side	+	watch	+	D
water	=	Right Back Side	+	water	+	D
wave	=	Right Back Side	+	wave	+	D
way	=	Right Back Side	+	way	+	D
we	=	Right Back Side	+	we	+	D
wear	=	Right Back Side	+	wear	+	D
weather	=	Right Back Side	+	weather	+	D
week	=	Right Back Side	+	week	+	D
weight	=	Right Back Side	+	weight	+	D
well	=	Right Back Side	+	well	+	D
went	=	Right Back Side	+	went	+	D
were	=	Right Back Side	+	were	+	D
west	=	Right Back Side	+	west	+	D
what	=	Right Back Side	+	what	+	D
wheel	=	Right Back Side	+	wheel	+	D
when	=	Right Back Side	+	when	+	D

whether	=	Right Back Side	+	whether	+	D
which	=	Right Back Side	+	which	+	D
while	=	Right Back Side	+	while	+	D
white	=	Right Back Side	+	white	+	D
whole	=	Right Back Side	+	whole	+	D
whose	=	Right Back Side	+	whose	+	D
why	=	Right Back Side	+	why	+	D
wide	=	Right Back Side	+	wide	+	D
wife	=	Left Back Side	+	wife	+	D
wild	=	Right Back Side	+	wild	+	D
will	=	Right Back Side	+	will	+	D
win	=	Right Back Side	+	win	+	D
wind	=	Right Back Side	+	wind	+	D
window	=	Right Back Side	+	window	+	D
wing	=	Right Back Side	+	wing	+	D
winter	=	Right Back Side	+	winter	+	D
wire	=	Right Back Side	+	wire	+	D
wish	=	Right Back Side	+	wish	+	D

with	=	Right Back Side	+	with	+ D
women	=	Left Back Side	+	women	+ D
wonder	=	Right Back Side	+	wonder	+ D
won't	=	Right Back Side	+	won't	+ D
wood	=	Right Back Side	+	wood	+ D
word	=	Right Back Side	+	word	+ D
work	=	Right Back Side	+	work	+ D
world	=	Right Back Side	+	world	+ D
would	=	Right Back Side	+	would	+ D
write	=	Right Back Side	+	write	+ D
written	=	Right Back Side	+	written	+ D
wrong	=	Right Back Side	+	wrong	+ D
wrote	=	Right Back Side	+	wrote	+ D
Yard	=	Right Back Side	+	Yard	+ D
Year	=	Right Back Side	+	Year	+ D
Yellow	=	Right Back Side	+	Yellow	+ D
Yes	=	Right Back Side	+	Yes	+ D
Yet	=	Right Back Side	+	Yet	+ D

You	=	Right Back Side	+	You	+	D
Young	=	Left Back Side	+	Young	+	D
Your	=	Right Back Side	+	Your	+	D

A New Era.
Visit www.twofuture.world

Signed
David Gomadza
The First Global President of the World
11/04/203
ifo@twofuture.world
00447719210295

www.ingramcontent.com/pod-product-compliance
Lightning Source LLC
Chambersburg PA
CBHW021829170526
45157CB00007B/2738